HOW YOUR EATING HABITS AFFECTS YOUR SKIN

TIPS FOR NOURISHING YOUR SKIN WITH DIET

AHMED .R

Contents

CHAPTER ONE

INTRODUCTION

Your food choices have a big impact on your skin's health and appearance in addition to your general health. In terms of skincare, the adage "you are what you eat" is accurate. Food has an effect on many skin issues, ranging from dryness and aging to acne and inflammation.

We'll look at how your eating habits impact your skin in this guide, and why choosing wholesome foods is essential to keeping your complexion looking good. We'll explore the science underlying the connection between skin health and diet, common dietary components that affect skin disorders, and doable advice for mindful eating that will promote clear, bright, and youthful-looking skin.

Knowing how your food choices affect your skin can help you make more informed decisions about your skincare routine and nutrition, which will result in healthier, more radiant skin from the inside out. Let's investigate the intriguing relationship that exists between your eating habits and the health and beauty of your skin.

Diet is important for healthy skin

It is impossible to exaggerate the significance of diet for healthy skin. The building blocks and nutrients required to maintain the function, look, and health of your skin are found in the foods you eat. Why diet is important for healthy skin

Delivery of Nutrients: Dietary nutrients are necessary for the development, maintenance, and regeneration of skin cells. Essential nutrients that maintain skin health and function include vitamins, minerals, antioxidants, and fatty acids.

Hydration: Sustaining skin suppleness and wetness requires enough hydration. Drinking enough water and eating meals high in moisture helps maintain the skin's internal moisture levels, which lowers the likelihood of flakiness, dullness, and dryness.

Production of Collagen: Collagen is a structural protein that gives skin its suppleness and strength. Collagen synthesis depends on a number of substances, including antioxidants, amino acids, and vitamin C. Consuming meals high in collagen can help maintain the firmness and suppleness of your skin.

Protection from Environmental Damage: The antioxidants in fruits, vegetables, and other plant-based foods assist in shielding the skin from the damaging effects of oxidative stress brought on by pollutants, UV rays, and other environmental contaminants. Free radicals are countered by antioxidants, which lowers the chance of wrinkles, sun damage, and early aging.

Reduction of Inflammation: Psoriasis, eczema, and acne are among the skin disorders that are linked to chronic inflammation. Eating foods high in omega-3 fatty acids, nuts, seeds, and leafy greens can help lower inflammation and encourage healthier, clearer skin.

Oil Production Regulation: The skin's natural oil, sebum, can be regulated with the use of a balanced diet. Overproduction of sebum can result in acne, plugged pores, and greasy skin. Eating a diet high in zinc, vitamin A, and omega-3 fatty acids will help balance oil production and stop breakouts.

The gut-skin axis is the term for the relationship that is emerging research reveals exists between skin and gut health. Skin disorders like eczema, rosacea, and acne may be ameliorated by eating a balanced diet that promotes intestinal integrity and variety of the gut flora.

Wound Healing: Skin restoration and wound healing depend on a number of minerals, including zinc, vitamin C, protein, and vitamin A. Eating meals high in these nutrients can help cuts, scratches, and other skin injuries heal more quickly.

Overall, encouraging healthy, glowing skin requires a diet that is both nutritious and well-balanced. You may provide your skin the vital nutrients it requires to flourish by including a range of nutritious meals, such as fruits, vegetables, whole grains, lean proteins, and healthy fats. Reduced intake of processed meals, sugary snacks, and excessive alcohol use can also help preserve skin health and delay the aging process. Recall that proper nutrition of your body with the correct foods promotes good skin health is the foundation of skincare, which goes beyond topical treatments.

Recognizing How Diet Affects Skin Health

Maintaining a healthy and bright complexion requires an understanding of how diet affects skin health. Your diet has a direct impact on several areas of skin health, such as appearance, aging, inflammation, and moisture. How food affects skin health is as follows:

Hydration: Sustaining skin suppleness and wetness requires proper hydration. Eating and drinking hydrating meals and drinks, like fruits and vegetables high in water content, keeps the skin hydrated from the inside out. On the other hand, dehydrated skin might appear flaky, dry, and lifeless due to a diet low in water.

Nutrient Intake: Food-based nutrients are essential for maintaining the health and function of the skin. The building blocks required for skin cell growth, repair, and regeneration are found in fruits, vegetables, whole grains, lean proteins, and healthy fats. These include vitamins, minerals, antioxidants, and vital fatty acids.

Chronic inflammation is associated with a number of skin disorders, such as psoriasis, eczema, and acne. Inflammation can be exacerbated by certain dietary components, including processed foods, sugary snacks, and unhealthy fats. Conversely, eating foods high in antioxidants, such leafy greens, nuts, seeds, and fatty fish, can help lower inflammation and support healthier, clearer skin.

Antioxidant Protection: The skin is shielded from oxidative stress brought on by pollutants, UV rays, and other environmental variables by the antioxidants present in colored fruits, vegetables, and other plant-based diets. Free radicals are neutralized by antioxidants, minimizing cellular damage and lowering the chance of wrinkles, UV damage, and early aging.

Production of Collagen: Collagen is a structural protein that gives skin its suppleness and strength. Collagen formation requires certain nutrients, including antioxidants, amino acids, and vitamin C. Consuming foods high in collagen, such as leafy greens, berries, citrus fruits, and bone broth, can help maintain firmer skin and lessen the appearance of wrinkles.

Oil Balance: The natural oil on the skin, sebum, can be affected by diet. Eating a diet high in zinc, vitamin A, and omega-3 fatty acids helps control oil production and prevents excessive sebum production, which lowers the likelihood of acne outbreaks, clogged pores, and oily skin.

Gut Health: A new body of research refers to this relationship as the "gut-skin axis" between skin and gut health. Skin disorders like eczema, rosacea, and acne may be ameliorated by eating a balanced diet that promotes intestinal integrity and variety of the gut flora.

You can nourish your skin from the inside out by being aware of how diet affects the health of your skin and choosing foods carefully. Maintaining skin health as you age can be achieved by consuming a range of nutrient-dense foods, drinking plenty of water, reducing inflammatory and processed foods, and encouraging a clear, radiant complexion.

The Essential Nutrients for Skin Health

Several nutrients are necessary to keep skin in good condition. These nutrients are essential for maintaining the structure, hydration, repair, and general appearance of the skin. The following are some vital nutrients that are necessary for good skin health:

Vitamin C: Packed with antioxidant properties, vitamin C promotes the synthesis of collagen, keeping skin supple and tight. It also lessens inflammation, speeds up the healing of wounds, and shields the skin from UV ray damage. Broccoli, bell peppers, strawberries, kiwi, and citrus fruits are all great sources of vitamin C.

Another strong antioxidant that helps shield the skin from oxidative damage brought on by free radicals is vitamin E. It may also aid in lessening the visibility of wrinkles and scars while promoting skin hydration and healing. Rich sources of vitamin E include avocado, spinach, nuts, seeds, and vegetable oils.

Vitamin A: Vitamin A is essential for the development, maintenance, and regeneration of skin cells. It supports the skin's natural moisture barrier, encourages the formation of collagen, and aids in the maintenance of healthy skin tissues. Vitamin A-rich foods include liver, sweet potatoes, carrots, spinach, and kale.

Omega-3 Fatty Acids: These important fats support the integrity of the skin barrier, lower inflammation, and keep the skin hydrated. Additionally, they lessen the chance of acne and other skin disorders by regulating oil production. Walnuts, chia seeds, flaxseeds, and fatty fish (sardines, mackerel, and salmon) are good sources of omega-3 fatty acids.

Zinc: This mineral is essential for both wound healing and healthy skin.

CHAPTER TWO

It boosts immunological response, lowers inflammation, and controls oil production. Skin conditions including eczema, acne, and slowed wound healing can be brought on by a zinc deficiency. Zinc-rich foods include oysters, steak, chicken, beans, nuts, and whole grains.

Selenium: This antioxidant mineral aids in shielding the skin from inflammation and oxidative damage. Additionally, it helps the thyroid, which has an indirect impact on skin health. Rich sources of selenium include eggs, whole grains, shellfish, chicken, and brazil nuts.

Vitamin B7, sometimes referred to as biotin, is necessary for strong, healthy skin, hair, and nails. It helps stop dryness, irritation, and rashes while promoting the growth and repair of skin cells. Skin conditions such as dermatitis can result from a lack of biotin. Good sources of biotin include eggs, sweet potatoes, nuts, seeds, and spinach.

Collagen Peptides: Collagen is a protein that helps keep the skin tight and supple by giving it structural support. Collagen peptides are readily absorbed forms of collagen that can be found in collagen-rich foods including fish, chicken skin soup, and supplements.

Including a range of foods high in nutrients in your diet can assist guarantee that you are receiving the necessary nutrients for radiant, healthy skin. Further supporting skin health and maintaining a youthful appearance are drinking plenty of water, limiting UV exposure, and adopting good skincare practices. For individualized advice, speak with a medical practitioner or qualified dietitian if you have any particular skin issues or deficiencies.

Sugar's Relationship to Skin Health

There is a complex relationship between sugar and skin health, with too much sugar having a variety of detrimental consequences on the skin. Sugar may have the following effects on skin health:

Glycation: Dangerous chemicals known as advanced glycation end products (AGEs) are created when blood sugar molecules bind to skin proteins including collagen and elastin. Because AGEs cause collagen and elastin fibers to cross-link and harden, they contribute to the aging of the skin by creating wrinkles, sagging, and a loss of skin suppleness.

Inflammation: Consuming large amounts of sugar can cause inflammation in the skin as well as other parts of the body. Numerous skin disorders, including rosacea, psoriasis, eczema, and acne, are associated with chronic inflammation. Inflammation can exacerbate pre-existing skin disorders and be a contributing factor to irritation, edema, and redness.

Acne Formation: Eating foods high in glucose, which quickly elevate blood sugar, might cause hormonal changes and enhance the skin's sebum production. Bacteria, dead skin cells, and excess sebum can block pores and cause acne outbreaks. Research has indicated that diets heavy in sugar and processed carbs are linked to a higher chance of developing acne.

Skin Aging: Sugar consumption can hasten the aging process of the skin by encouraging oxidative stress and the breakdown of collagen. An imbalance between the body's antioxidants and free radicals causes oxidative stress, which damages cells and accelerates aging. Furthermore, sugar has the potential to weaken the body's built-in antioxidant defenses, which can exacerbate oxidative damage and lead to wrinkles, fine lines, and uneven skin tone.

Dehydration: Consuming a lot of sugar can cause dehydration because the blood sugar's excess pulls water from cells, especially skin cells. Dehydrated skin is more prone to wrinkles and fine lines because it looks parched, dry, and less plump. Maintaining skin moisture and fostering a healthy complexion depend on proper hydration.

Skin Conditions: Consuming a lot of sugar can make some skin conditions worse, such psoriasis and eczema. Sugar has the ability to cause the body to respond inflammatoryly, exacerbating symptoms and producing itching, redness, and discomfort.

Gut-Skin Connection: A growing body of research points to a connection, or gut-skin axis, between skin and intestinal health. Sugar- and processed-food-rich diets can upset the balance of the gut bacteria, causing inflammation and skin problems. Skin issues may improve if gut health is improved through dietary changes, such as cutting back on sweets and eating more fiber-rich foods.

Overall, maintaining skin health and lowering the risk of skin problems and early aging can be achieved by cutting back on sugar intake and choosing a balanced diet full of whole foods, fruits, vegetables, lean meats, and healthy fats. In addition, hydration, stress management, and adhering to proper skincare practices are crucial for glowing, clean skin.

Skin Hydration Is Essential

Since it is essential to preserving the skin's overall health, function, and attractiveness, hydration is vital for skin health. This is why skin needs to be properly hydrated:

Moisture Barrier: The stratum corneum, the outermost layer of skin, serves as a barrier to keep moisture in and shield the body from viruses, toxins, and environmental irritants. Sufficient hydration contributes to the integrity of this moisture barrier and keeps the skin robust, supple, and moisturized.

Skin Elasticity: The skin's capacity to stretch and return to its natural form is referred to as skin elasticity, and it is influenced by hydration.

Dehydrated skin can look dull, dry, and more prone to fine lines and wrinkles. In contrast, well-hydrated skin looks plump, firm, and youthful.

Nutrient Transport: Staying properly hydrated helps skin cells absorb and use oxygen and nutrients, which supports the growth, repair, and regeneration of skin cells. Bloodstream nutrients promote the skin's health, vigor, and ability to fend off environmental damage and oxidative stress. They nourish the skin from the inside out.

Elimination of Toxins: Drinking enough water encourages the body to expel waste and toxins through perspiration and sweat. Toxins are effectively removed from the body when it is well hydrated, which lowers the likelihood of skin conditions like acne, inflammation, and dullness.

Temperature Regulation: Sweating allows the skin to release heat, which is essential for controlling body temperature. Maintaining the ideal body temperature requires adequate hydration to avoid overheating and perspiration, both of which can cause dehydration and skin irritation.

Healing of Wounds: Skin restoration and wound healing depend on hydration. In addition to hastening the healing process and lowering the danger of infection and scarring, moisture encourages the growth of new skin cells. Wounds should be kept clean and moisturized to promote the best possible healing and reduce problems.

pH Balance: The skin naturally has a slightly acidic pH balance (around 5.5), which is maintained by hydration. Maintaining the integrity and health of the skin, avoiding microbial proliferation, and strengthening the protective layer of the skin all depend on a pH level that is balanced.

Prevention of Skin disorders: Dry, flaky, itchy, irritated, and inflammatory skin disorders are more likely to occur in dehydrated skin. You can lessen your risk of developing these problems and preserve a comfortable, healthy skin barrier by drinking enough water.

Drinking enough water throughout the day and include hydrating items like fruits, vegetables, soups, and herbal teas in your diet are vital ways to maintain proper hydration. Furthermore, humectants, emollients, and occlusives included in moisturizers and skincare products can help seal in moisture and preserve skin hydration levels. In general, encouraging healthy, glowing skin and bolstering general wellbeing need giving adequate attention to hydration.

Protein's Function in Skin Health

Protein is essential for preserving the health and vigor of the skin. The skin, which is the biggest organ in the body, depends on proteins for a number of structural, functional, and defensive purposes. Here's how protein supports healthy skin:

Production of Collagen: The skin's most prevalent protein, collagen is necessary to keep the skin's suppleness, firmness, and structure. Collagen helps to keep wrinkles and sagging by giving the skin's extracellular matrix structural stability. Foods high in protein supply the amino acids required for the synthesis of collagen, promoting healthy aging of the skin and reducing the visibility of fine lines and wrinkles.

Elastin Formation: The elasticity and resilience of skin are attributed to elastin, another structural protein. The skin may expand and revert to its natural form thanks to elastin fibers, which also keep the skin tight and prevent drooping.

Consuming protein helps elastin develop, which promotes suppleness and a youthful appearance of the skin.

Healing of Wounds: Tissue repair and wound healing depend on protein. The body needs amino acids from food protein after trauma or injury to repair damaged skin tissues and encourage the growth of new skin cells. Consuming enough protein promotes quicker wound healing, lessens scarring, and improves skin regeneration.

Immune function: The skin acts as a shield to keep the body safe from pollutants, infections, and environmental irritants. Protein is required to sustain immunological function and preserve the integrity of the skin. Antimicrobial peptides, cytokines, and immunoglobulins are a few examples of proteins that support the skin's defense against oxidative stress, inflammation, and infections.

Hydration and Moisture Retention: Proteins are important for preserving the moisture balance and hydration of the skin. A few proteins, like aquaporins and filaggrin, control the flow of water in the skin and contribute to ideal levels of hydration. Consuming enough protein maintains the integrity of the skin's barrier, avoiding dehydration and fostering a radiant complexion.

Antioxidant Protection: Certain proteins have the ability to neutralize free radicals and shield the skin from oxidative damage by acting as antioxidants. Wrinkles, skin problems, and premature aging are all influenced by oxidative stress. Antioxidants included in diets high in protein promote skin health and lower the risk of oxidative damage.

Health of Hair and Nails: Proteins are necessary to keep hair and nails healthy and intact. The fibrous protein keratin, which is present in hair and nails, gives them resistance, strength, and structure. Consuming enough protein encourages the body to produce keratin, which in turn promotes healthy hair development and guards against split ends, brittleness, and breaking.

Including foods high in protein in your diet, such as fish, chicken, eggs, dairy products, legumes, nuts, seeds, and soy products, will help maintain the health and vitality of your skin. Furthermore, as protein is necessary for many physiological functions other than skin health, eating enough of it is crucial for general health and wellbeing. For individualized advice catered to your requirements, speak with a medical practitioner or qualified dietitian if you have certain skin issues or dietary limitations.

CHAPTER THREE

Healthy Fats' Impact on Skin

Healthy fats are essential for preserving the health of the skin and fostering a glowing complexion. Including sufficient levels of good fats in your diet can improve your skin in a number of ways. The following are a few of the main ways that healthy fats benefit skin health:

Moisture Retention: Good fats contribute to the preservation of the skin's natural lipid barrier, which shields the skin from outside aggressors and keeps moisture from evaporating from it. By maintaining the skin's moisture, suppleness, and softness, its barrier function lowers the likelihood of dryness, flakiness, and rough texture.

Skin Elasticity: To preserve skin elasticity, essential fatty acids like omega-3 and omega-6 fatty acids are essential. These lipids aid in the synthesis of skin lipids, which preserve the flexibility and structural integrity of the skin. Increased elasticity can make the skin appear smoother and younger by minimizing the appearance of fine lines and wrinkles.

Reduction of Inflammation: The anti-inflammatory qualities of healthy fats can aid in the reduction of skin inflammation. Skin diseases like psoriasis, eczema, and acne are linked to chronic inflammation. Particularly omega-3 fatty acids have been demonstrated to lower inflammatory markers in the skin, resulting in clearer, more tranquil skin as well as less redness and irritation.

Wound Healing: By supplying vital nutrients and encouraging tissue repair, healthy fats aid in the skin's natural healing process. It has been demonstrated that omega-3 fatty acids in particular can limit scarring, reduce inflammation, and speed up the healing process from wounds. You may speed up the healing process for cuts, scratches, and other skin injuries by include healthy fats in your diet.

Protection from UV Damage: The photoprotective qualities of certain healthy fats, such the polyphenols and antioxidants present in plant-based oils, can aid in shielding the skin from UV ray damage. These lipids lower the risk of sunburn, early aging, and skin cancer by neutralizing free radicals produced by UV light. Although they can't take the place of sunscreen, good fats can enhance skin health overall and support attempts to protect the sun.

Nutrition for Hair and Nails: Good fats are important for keeping hair and nails looking and feeling good. The natural oil produced by the skin, sebum, which hydrates the scalp and hair follicles and lessens dryness and brittleness, is supported by essential fatty acids. You may encourage strong, healthy nails and glossy, lustrous hair by include healthy fats in your diet.

Avocados, nuts and seeds (including chia, walnut, and almond seeds), fatty fish (such salmon, mackerel, and sardines), olive, coconut, and flaxseed oils are good sources of healthful fats. You may maintain overall skin health and vibrancy and offer necessary nutrients by including a range of these healthy fats in your diet. For best results, always remember to include them in a balanced diet and consume them in moderation.

A number of foods are recognized for their ability to support skin health by offering vital nutrients, antioxidants, and hydration. By include these foods in your diet, you can support a beautiful complexion and nourish your skin from the inside out. The following foods are known to support healthy skin:

Fatty Fish: Rich in omega-3 fatty acids, fatty fish like salmon, mackerel, and sardines support skin hydration, suppleness, and barrier function. Additionally, omega-3s contain anti-inflammatory qualities that help lower the chance of developing psoriasis, dermatitis, and acne.

Avocados: Rich in antioxidants, vitamins, and good fats that nourish the skin, avocados are a superfood. They include vitamin C, which encourages collagen formation and skin regeneration, monounsaturated fats, which help retain skin hydration, and vitamin E, which guards against oxidative damage.

Nuts and Seeds: Rich in important fatty acids, vitamins, minerals, and antioxidants, nuts and seeds including almonds, walnuts, flaxseeds, and chia seeds are a great source of nutrition. These nutrients defend against UV rays and inflammation while also promoting skin hydration, suppleness, and barrier function.

Fruits: A lot of fruits are good for your skin because they're high in water, vitamins, minerals, and antioxidants. Antioxidants found in berries, especially raspberries, blueberries, and strawberries, help shield the skin from oxidative stress and early aging. Vitamin C, which is abundant in citrus fruits like oranges, lemons, and grapefruits, encourages the formation of collagen and brightens the skin.

Vegetables: Rich in vitamins, minerals, antioxidants, and phytonutrients that promote skin health are colorful vegetables. Vitamins A, C, and E are abundant in leafy greens like spinach, kale, and Swiss chard; these nutrients support skin hydration, repair, and protection. Beta-carotene, found in abundance in bell peppers, sweet potatoes, and carrots, is converted by the body into vitamin A and promotes healthy skin.

Green Tea: Packed with antioxidants, polyphenols, and catechins, green tea helps shield the skin from sun damage, inflammation, and early aging. Regular consumption of green tea can enhance skin tone, lessen inflammation and redness, and improve the health of the skin overall.

Olive Oil: Rich in monounsaturated fats, antioxidants, and vitamins E and K, extra virgin olive oil is a healthy fat. It lessens inflammation, nourishes and moisturizes the skin, and shields it from oxidative harm. Your skin can benefit from consuming olive oil topically as a moisturizer and by including it in your diet.

Probiotic Foods: Rich in helpful bacteria, foods high in probiotics, such as yogurt, kefir, sauerkraut, and kimchi, boost digestive health and may help alleviate skin disorders including rosacea, eczema, and acne. Immune system and general skin health depend on a healthy gut microbiota.

By include a range of these nutrient-dense, skin-friendly foods in your diet, you can support a healthy, glowing complexion and nourish your skin. In order to maintain general skin health and stay hydrated, don't forget to drink lots of water throughout the day. To further promote ideal skin health, have a balanced diet high in whole foods and low in processed foods, sweets, and alcohol.

Foods That Could Make Skin Conditions Worse

There is evidence that some diets can exacerbate a number of skin diseases, such as rosacea, psoriasis, eczema, and acne. Although individual triggers may differ, the following popular meals may worsen skin conditions:

Dairy Products: Consuming dairy products, particularly cow's milk, has been linked to a higher chance of developing acne. Hormones found in milk, such as insulin-like growth factor 1 (IGF-1), may increase the production of sebum and cause clogged pores and acne outbreaks. Dairy products can also exacerbate pre-existing skin diseases like psoriasis and eczema in certain people by inducing inflammation and immunological responses.

Foods with a high glycemic index (GI) include processed carbs, white bread, white rice, sweet snacks, and sugar. These foods can cause insulin surges and sharp increases in blood sugar levels. Increased sebum production, inflammation, and acne development may be triggered by elevated insulin levels. Eating a diet rich in high-GI foods has been linked to a higher chance of developing acne.

Sugary Foods and Drinks: Sugary foods and drinks, such as sodas, sweets, pastries, and snacks with added sugar, can cause oxidative stress, insulin resistance, and inflammation in the body. Consuming too much sugar can impede wound healing, exacerbate acne, and age the skin more quickly. Furthermore, eating sugary food might upset the gut microbiota's equilibrium, which may have an indirect impact on skin health.

Fried and Greasy meals: Fried and greasy meals are heavy in calories and bad fats. Examples of these foods are french fries, potato chips, fried chicken, and fast food. Overindulging in fatty and fried foods can aggravate acne and cause oxidative stress and inflammation. Furthermore, eating greasy meals might make acne outbreaks worse by aggravating oily skin and blocked pores.

Foods containing gluten: Foods containing gluten, such as wheat, barley, and rye, can cause autoimmune reactions and inflammatory reactions in people with celiac disease or gluten sensitivity. Ingestion of gluten can cause skin problems like dermatitis herpetiformis, a type of rash that is sensitive to gluten. For those with gluten-related skin issues, cutting less on gluten-containing foods may help improve their skin symptoms.

Spicy meals: Capsaicin, a substance that can induce flushing, redness, and irritation in sensitive people, is found in spicy meals including hot peppers, chili, and curry. Eating spicy food might worsen the symptoms of rosacea and cause more redness and inflammation in those who have sensitive skin.

Alcohol: Drinking too much alcohol can cause the body to become dehydrated, which can result in dry, dull skin. Additionally, alcohol causes blood vessels to dilate and increases blood flow to the skin's surface, which aggravates rosacea symptoms and causes facial flushing. Furthermore, drinking alcohol can cause hormonal imbalances and impairments to the liver, which may exacerbate acne and other skin disorders.

It's crucial to remember that different people may have different triggers, and not everyone will be negatively impacted by these meals. Consider keeping a food diary and consulting a medical expert or certified nutritionist to identify and remove potential triggers from your diet if you believe that certain foods are aggravating your skin issue. A balanced, nutrient-rich diet and dietary adjustments can assist to enhance skin health and lessen the severity of skin disorders.

Customizing Your Food to Improve Your Skin Health

Identifying your unique skin difficulties, comprehending potential food triggers, and making educated decisions to support optimal skin function and appearance are all part of customizing your diet for better skin health. The following actions can help you customize your diet for healthier skin:

Determine Skin Concerns: Make a note of any particular issues you may be having with your skin, such as rosacea, eczema, acne, dryness, or early aging. Think about any possible triggers you've seen, such as particular foods, drinks, or environmental conditions, as well as when your symptoms go better or worse.

Maintain a Food Journal: Maintain a thorough food journal to monitor any changes in your skin's condition as well as your nutritional consumption. Keep track of the items you consume, the amounts you eat, the times you eat, and any symptoms or skin responses you encounter. This might assist you in determining patterns and possible food triggers associated with the health of your skin.

Remove Possible Triggers: Take into consideration removing any dietary triggers that can make your skin issues worse, based on your food diary and observations. Dairy products, foods high on the glycemic index, sugary snacks, fried and greasy foods, gluten-containing cereals, spicy foods, and alcohol are examples of common triggers.

Emphasis on Nutrient-Rich Foods: Give top priority to foods high in nutrients that promote good skin, such as fruits, vegetables, whole grains, legumes, lean meats, and healthy fats. These foods supply vital vitamins, minerals, antioxidants, and omega-3 fatty acids that support a healthy complexion and nourish the skin from the inside out.

Eat Foods High in Skin-Friendly Nutrients: Eat foods high in skin-friendly nutrients that address the particular issues you are having with your skin. For instance, diets rich in zinc, omega-3 fatty acids, vitamin C, and vitamin E can help produce collagen, lower inflammation, and encourage skin hydration and repair.

Stay Hydrated: To maintain skin hydration and suppleness, sip lots of water throughout the day. You can also encourage good skin hydration by include hydrating foods like fruits and vegetables, coconut water, and herbal teas in your regular fluid consumption.

Handle Stress: Stress can aggravate skin disorders and lead to oxidative stress and inflammation in the body. Engage in stress-relieving activities that enhance general skin health and encourage relaxation, such as yoga, deep breathing exercises, meditation, and outdoor time.

Seek Professional Advice: If you're unclear about how to treat particular skin conditions or which dietary adjustments to make, think considering consulting a dermatologist, allergist, or registered dietitian. They can offer tailored advice depending on your particular requirements, medical background, and skin type.

Through customized nutrition planning, you may nourish your skin from the inside out and encourage a healthy, beautiful complexion. To maximize your skin health and general wellbeing, pay attention to how your body reacts to various foods and lifestyle circumstances. Then, make modifications as necessary.

Summary

In conclusion, it is clear that the condition and look of your skin are greatly influenced by the foods you eat. The vital vitamins, minerals, antioxidants, and healthy fats required to preserve skin moisture, suppleness, and general wellbeing can be obtained from a diet that is well-balanced and nutrient-rich. On the other hand, unhealthful eating habits, such ingesting large amounts of sugar, fats, and processed foods, can lead to oxidative stress, inflammation, and skin disorders like eczema, acne, and early aging.

You can maintain ideal skin health and encourage a glowing complexion by forming good eating habits and making wise dietary choices. This entails drinking enough of water, limiting your intake of substances that may irritate or trigger your skin, and include a range of fruits, vegetables, lean meats, whole grains, and healthy fats in your diet. A comprehensive approach to skin health also includes following healthy skincare practices, getting enough sleep, and controlling stress.

Keep in mind that each individual has a different type of skin, so what suits one person may not suit another. It's critical to listen to your body's signals, keep an eye on how your skin reacts to certain diets and lifestyle choices, and, if necessary, seek professional advice. You can take care of your skin from the inside out and keep a healthy, radiant complexion for years to come by being proactive with your food and skincare routine.

THE END